# HIGH INTENSITY KETTLEBELL FITNESS

*Complete Guide to Super Fitness in 20 Minutes or Less*

## MICHAEL STEFANO

# TABLE OF CONTENTS

## ACE STUDY

BENEFITS OF KETTLEBELLS

The American Council on Exercise (ACE), America's Workout Watchdog, enlisted the research experts at the University of Wisconsin-La Crosse's department of Exercise and Sport Science to conduct a study led by John Porcari, Ph.D. The research team recruited 30 healthy, relatively fit male and female volunteers. The subjects were randomly divided into two groups. Eighteen volunteers (9 male, 9 female) were put into the experimental group, while 12 others (6 male, 6 female) were used as the control group. Twice weekly the subjects participated in kettlebell training. At the beginning of the study, the trainers encouraged participants to use a weight that felt manageable and then progress to heavier kettlebells as they felt more comfortable with the movements.

In addition to the *predictable* strength gains, kettlebell training was also shown to *markedly increase aerobic capacit*y, *improve dynamic balance* and *dramatically increase core strength*. "When most people think of resistance training, they don't think of being able to increase the aerobic capacity," says Dr. John Porcari, "Yet, we saw a 13.8 percent increase in aerobic capacity." The most dramatic increase in strength came in abdominal core strength, which was boosted by 70 percent. "Kettlebell training increases strength, which you'd expect, but you also get these other benefits," says Porcari. "You don't really do resistance training expecting to get an aerobic capacity benefit, and you don't do resistance training and expect to improve your core strength, unless of course you're specifically doing core-strengthening exercises. But with kettlebells you're able to get a wide variety of benefits with one pretty intense workout."

The bottom line is, kettlebells may be decidedly old school, but thanks to the explosive, total-body nature of kettlebell training, its potential for serious body benefits are just as strong as ever. "It's a hell great workout, but you really need to get proper instruction before you do it," says Porcari. "Good form is key to avoiding injury." Get a minimum of two to three training sessions with a certified instructor. Consider using a workout video to follow along with for proper form.

## ABOUT THE AUTHOR

Michael Stefano, FDNY retired Captain, is the author of *The Firefighter's Workout Book©* (The Train-For-Life Program for Men and Women), functional fitness expert, and HIKF Master Coach, as well as a Master Coach with the World Kettlebell Club, having studied directly with kettlebell lifting World Champion, *Valery Fedorenko*. Mike is also an American Council on Exercise certified instructor and creator of the High Intensity Kettlebell Fitness Program. Currently, Mike owns and operates KBNY, a full time kettlebell gymnasium on Long Island, New York.

*"Mike Stefano has been instrumental in the development of World Kettlebell Club and its subsidiaries and offshoots such as the American Kettlebell Club, as well as the creation of AKC Fitness. He also has helped create the First Responder PROTOCOL, marking a monumental change in the preparedness of Firefighters and other Emergency Responders around the world. I have no hesitation recommending Coach Stefano."* **– kettlebell world champion, *Valery Fedorenko***

# INTRODUCTION

Kettlebell lifting, as a sport or fitness system, has been around for a long time – some say centuries in Russia. But the greatest benefits lie in the traditional Russian lifts that are covered in great detail in this book. The kettlebell is moved with *fully body explosive*, yet *smooth* and *fluid movements*. Think ballet meets Olympic weight lifting. The true kettlebell lifter, over time, will develop not only android levels of strength, endurance and power, while learning how to relax between repetitions, but split second timing, honing the central nervous system, a benefit that crosses over to many other activities

Sets are performed for time versus just a rep count. Reps are tracked and used as one of the ways to control intensity (along with six other variables discussed in detail later in this manual). The lifter must learn to move "with" the kettlebell, striving for total efficiency, thereby generating tremendous force while avoiding injury. And it doesn't end there. Technique, efficiency, performance continue to sky rocket, while the body acclimates and adapts.

## 8 MAJOR BENEFITS OF

## KETTLEBELL FITNESS

1. **MULTI-DIMENSIONAL:** BUILDS STRENGTH AND ENDURANCE SIMULTANEOUSLY

2. **BODY SCULPTER:** TONES, DEFINES LEGS, UPPER BODY, AND CORE

3. **TOTAL BODY**: CONDITIONG: SUPERIOR FULL BODY CONDITIONING TOOL

4. **POSTERIOR CHAIN:** WORKS THE HARD TO REACH "POSTERIOR CHAIN"

5. **USER FRIENDLY:** SAFE, EFFECTIVE, AND EASY TO LEARN

6. **FLEXIBLE:** CAN BE INCORPORATED INTO ANY OTHER WORKOUT

7. **PRACTICAL:** MINIMAL EQUIPMENT SPACE, AND TIME REQUIRED

8. **HIGHLY CALORIC:** CONSISTENTLY EFFECTIVE AT BURNING FAT

## HOW TO USE THIS BOOK

First carefully read through Part I, *Program Overview*, as this gives the reader a general overview of the evolution of the program. In Part II, *Mastering Kettlebell Technique*, you'll get right to work. Some are visual learners, while others do better with the verbal or written word. Either way watch the video (live links), then read through each exercise, one lift at a time. If possible, you should be working with a professional grade or competition kettlebell for best results. Opt for a light weight to start, typically 10kg for women and 12kg for men, but pro-grade kettlebells are now being produced as light as 4kg. *Be sure you work as light as necessary to remain in total control of the kettlebell, so as to avoid injury.* It's a good idea to begin with the Initial *12-Step Progression* (see Part II), as you build skill, strength, and endurance, while you gradually digest the rest of the information in this manual. Continue to practice, workout, and master technique in the various lifts. Once you can handle 20 minute non-stop sets, you can select from just about any PROTOCOL that's listed in Part III, using the HIKF *Seven Variables on Intensity* to adjust the workout to your appropriate level.

# I: PROGRAM OVERVIEW

**High Intensity Kettlebell Fitness**

Welcome to the *High Intensity Kettlebell Fitness eBook*, where you can achieve real results in how you look, feel, and perform, **while avoiding injury**. At Gym KBNY, we utilize this exact same system, and put tremendous focus on *execution of proper form and technique*, as the ultimate protection against the endless set back of injures that plague most fitness enthusiasts

While it's hard to pin down an exact date, some say Kettlebell lifting has been around for centuries, becoming a competitive sport in Russia in 1948. Since then, *Kettlebell Sport Athletes* have worked relentlessly at perfecting technique with *competitive* lifts. This high level skill has been continually refined, and passed down from *coach to athlete* from *generation to generation* – but without much written documentation. This sophisticated and somewhat technical approach to kettlebell lifting was popularized in the United States in 2007, with the formation of the American Kettlebell Club® by world champion lifter, *Valery Fedorenko*, considered by some to be the world's foremost authority on kettlebells. The *High Intensity Kettlebell Fitness*® eBook will provide the reader with not only the detailed knowledge behind this ancient system, but the specific methodology necessary to progress at every levels.

As a New York City firefighter, fitness author and instructor, I've always been drawn to the more functional aspect of physical conditioning as a way to keep the body in peek physical condition, and ready for anything – but I've always stuck by the golden rule of, *do no harm*. My strategy is to recreate appropriate intensity, so as to produce *verifiable, repeatable results*, but *without unnecessary injury*.

Back in 2006, I had only seen kettlebells online and in magazines, but lacked any firsthand experience with a true expert. After some extensive research and some painful trial and error, I was introduced to world champion kettlebell lifter and record holder, *Valery Fedorenko,* and the *American Kettlebell Club*® (AKC). I applied for a position as the club's *Fire Rescue Advisor*, and was awarded the position. This gave me the unique opportunity to work side by side with an Honored Master of Sport (kettlebells highest ranking). After much trust, study, training, and dedication, I moved on to become a *Master Coach* with the World Kettlebell Club by the end of that same year (2007).

In the months and years that followed, I continued to work alongside Valery, assisting in over a dozen competitions, seminars, workshops and certifications. I worked closely with Coach Fedorenko at numerous AKC seminars, while at the same time, running my own kettlebell fitness gym. What I learned was priceless information and methodology, brand new on the American fitness scene.

On the home front, I immediately adapted and applied my newly found kettlebell coaching skills to both my firefighter and civilian clients. The consistently high level of physical conditioning and explosive force I was able to repeatedly produce in just about anyone who was willing to do the work was something I'd never experienced before.  As long as the lifter did the program, the results were ALWAYS there. Kettlebell lifting, in its purest form, has the potential to transform not only every individual who does the work, but dramatically change the way all Americans look at fitness.

Authentic kettlebells, sometimes described as a *running with weights*, employs the concept of *timed sets – picking up a kettlebell and not setting it down for up to 20 minutes or more*. This remarkably effective, and a surprisingly safe, and extremely sound system that is *forever repeatable*. It works with just about lifter, every time. Kettlebells, *when used correctly,* can easily be adapted to a wide variety of goals and fitness levels – with a statistically significant low rate of injury, even amongst the top lifters performing the most extreme sets.

Kettlebell champion, Valery Fedorenko, has passed this dynamic skill on to me. Over the last seven years, I've mastered the process of educating the American public on authentic kettlebell lifting. Whether for health, fitness, weight loss, explosive power, increased work capacity, competitive sports, or just warding off old age, *the system works*. I've had the unique privilege of working closely with hundreds of men and women locally, as well as with firefighters, athletes, and trainers from around the world via the internet and live seminars, certifications, and workshops. I've now developed my own dynamic system, steeped in authentic kettlebell technique, while making it work for the average American. The bottom line is BIG RESULTS. The *High Intensity Kettlebell Fitness* program will show the student, athlete and trainer how to achieve those same results.

Today, as an American Council on continuing education provider, kettlebell gym owner, and Master Coach and Trainer, I conduct kettlebell fitness seminars and workshops for firefighters, athletes, and trainers from around the world. *The High Intensity Kettlebell Fitness Program* are the culmination of years of training, and time-tested methodology, yet, this book is appropriate for every level kettlebell lifter, novice student to advanced athlete, seeking to use kettlebells and maximize results with minimal injury, as its main focus is teaching the proper technique behind each lift, the key to long lasting results.

## HIKF PROGRAM OBJECTIVES

1. Generate explosive, dynamic, yet fluid movements that produce little or no impact
2. Utilize timed sets where the kettlebell is lifted continuously for up to 20 minutes
3. Simultaneously build strength, power, muscular and cardiovascular endurance, and flexibility
4. Create a high caloric workload with every set (21 calories per minute according to studies)
5. Develop not only muscle, but strong and flexible, connective tissue for healthy joints
6. Safely and effectively develop appropriate programming for yourself or students

## TIMED SETS AND THE 7 VARIABLES

After my personal introduction to kettlebell lifting in late 2006, I recognized the benefits of this old-school, yet intelligent system, to functionally work the entire body, utilizing powerfully ballistic, yet totally fluid movement patterns, thus reducing the likelihood of acute or overuse injury that is usually associated with too much ballistic exercise. This proven methodology also came with a mega-high level of cardiovascular demand (potentially burning up to 21 calories per minute), as well as doing a stellar job at building strong, flexible muscles, joints and connective tissue.

Much like Kettlebell Sport training, the secret to the overall effectiveness of the HIKF system lies in its focus on *proper technique* coupled with *a high rep scheme*, and the primary emphasis on the *length of the set versus just a number of reps*. What makes the HIKF program work so well is the precise customization that's possible via the Seven Intensity Variables, and the inclusion of over 15PROVEN PROTOCOLs, which allow extremely high intensity levels to be reached, but with a relatively low risk of injury as you work with time tested routines. However, true success is only achieved with serious practice, and true proficiency with the core lifts, as well as a thorough understanding of the Seven Intensity Variables that make up the HIKF system. Kettlebell lifting is not meant to be mastered over a weekend course. This program manual is just your first baby step to getting to one of the most revolutionary, yet practical systems for developing overall strength, endurance, general conditioning, health, work capacity, coordination, explosiveness and athletic performance.

Unfortunately, quality kettlebell instruction is not so easy to find, due to the bastardization of the original sport methodology. HIKF technique is based on pure kettlebell sport methodology a taught to me directly by Valery Fedorenko. Most so-called kettlebell instruction winds up over simplified, and comes with no real track record. Perhaps the simplification attempts to ease the learning process, but unfortunately it lessens effectiveness. Much like a martial art, it's the purity of this authentic system that will win out in the long run and allow the student of High Intensity Kettlebell Fitness to rise above the rest. I've seen it personally happen dozens of times. The new student needs to be educated physically and mentally, and realize that performing a curl with a kettlebell is NOT true kettlebell fitness. Being able to exhibit proficiency with the core lifts presented in the next section will transform the novice lifter into stronger, leaner, more explosively powerful, kinesthetically self-aware and conditioned, human being.

## PROPER CLOTHING / ACCESSORIES

A cotton short-sleeved tee shirt provides the best protection for *catching* the kettlebell in the Rack position (as it's cleaned or dropped from Lockout). Opt for sweat pants or workout shorts that allow a full range of motion with no interference. Weight lifting shoes are considered to be the best footwear option, but a firm athletic shoe that offers good support, without too much cushion, is another sensible choice. Some form of forearm protection, such as sweat bands, ACE elastic wraps, or VF kettlebell shields are recommended, to absorb sweat and protect the forearms (available directly from the World Kettlebell Club). No gloves or hand protections should be worn, as this interferes with the kinesthetic awareness necessary to develop the proper feel (timing, coordination, control) with each exercise. If necessary to protect torn or blistered palms, a soft, thinned fabric (non-leather) glove can be worn with the fingers removed. Remember that the best protection against injury is proper timing, not protective gear.

## PAIN AND OVERUSE INJURIES

The new Kettlebell lifter will have a hard time discerning between healthy discomfort and dangerous pain. Typically, joint pain should not be tolerated, and a clear sign of a gross technique issue or simple overuse, but there is an acclimation period where the body will experience some pain no matter how perfect technique is. Any soreness that doesn't disappear in a day or two needs to be addressed, and you should see your health care professional if you feel you've sustained or aggravated an injury. But there is a lot that can be done to reduce injury. Kettlebell sets are hard, it hurts. There is no way around that. We seek to remove as much risk from the equation as possible. You'll find that lifter's with the best technique can perform the most extreme sets, with the least occurrence of injury. Kettlebell Sport includes some of the most intense all out performances in athletics today.

HIKF methodology enables the lifter to develop tremendous explosive force, but with the goal of a *soft* landing. Inflammation is the enemy, and learning to stop smoothly, on a dime every rep, is something that's perfected over time. Beginners should use every ache and pain as feedback on what needs to be fixed, where tension or inflammation may be building. *At higher intensities, avoiding injury is the key to success.* Early on, keep weight light to speed up the learning process, and not get hurt. At a certain point, when it comes time to jump to a heavier kettlebell, new mistakes will reveal themselves.  And sometimes this means going back to the drawing board. Look at this as an opportunity to remodel your home. Everything will be new and working perfectly once you get that new sheetrock up.

## MINOR INJURY / CAUSE CHART

DISCLAIMER: SEE YOUR DOCTOR FOR ALL SERIOIUS INJURIES

1. -Bruised Shoulder

    a. Improper Clean / Improper drop from Lockout

2. -Upper Trap Pain

    a. Over pulling the kettlebell with the arm during Swing, Clean, or Snatch

3. -Elbow Pain

    a. Bad timing when dropping the kettlebell from the Rack (Clean) or Lockout (Snatch)

4. -Bruised Forearm

    a. Maintaining a straight wrist in Rack and / or Lockout

5. -Wrist Pain

    a. Maintaining a straight wrist in Rack and / or Lockout

6. -Blistered Palm

    a. Squeezing the bell handle in Swing, Clean or Snatch / Not using the Fingerlock

7. -Low Back Pain

    a. Hyperextending (arch) or hyperflexing (round) the back during Swing, Clean, Snatch

8. -Hip Pain

    a. Allowing the hips to "crash" as the bell is pulled too hard in Swing, Clean or Snatch

9. -Knee Pain

    a. Bad timing in Push Press, Jerk, or LongCycle (first or second dip)

10. -Foot Pain

    a. Staying up on your toes (heels in the air) prior to launching the bell in

       Jerk or LongCycle

# II: MASTERING TECHNIQUE

Read the instructions listed with each lift as well as review the online video. The process of mastering true kettlebell technique doesn't happen overnight. As you educate your nervous system to move more efficiently, your body needs time to adapt to these new movement patterns. Be patient and practice, practice, practice. Proficient technique allows greater intensity levels, yet minimizes overuse injuries.

*I once asked Coach Fedorenko what he thought was the absolute best way to get good at Snatch. With an ingenious use of very few words, he simply answered, "Snatch". Makes perfect sense.*

## PROPER BREATHING

Initially it's important for the new lifter to learn the proper breathing pattern that's a big part of every lift. As a general rule, HIKF incorporates a *Yogic breathing style*, with no breath holds. In other words, whenever the spine flexes (as in forward bending – dropping the kettlebell), the lifter exhales, whenever the spine extends (as in back bending – bring the kettlebell to Rack or Lockout) the lifter inhales. Breathing during the static segment of each lift (Rack and Lockout) is not only permitted, but sometimes absolutely necessary. The lifter should use the breath to *orchestrate* each rep, improving coordination and timing, moving with the rhythm of the breath. The breath should be full, but not forced, through both the mouth and nose. Keeping your mouth open will ensure you never hold your breath (very important).   More specific instruction on the proper breathing pattern will be included with each lift.

## HOW TO ACCESS YOUR HIKF VIDEOS

Video goes a long was in demonstrating kettlebell technique, so instead of cluttering up these chapters with endless illustrations, I've made it easy for you to access free bonus video of all the lifts. Send an email with the words "**HIKF VIDEO**" in the subject line to: service@kbgym.com and you'll be sent an email with private links to all the HIKF exercise videos hosted on YouTube.

## 1: SWING

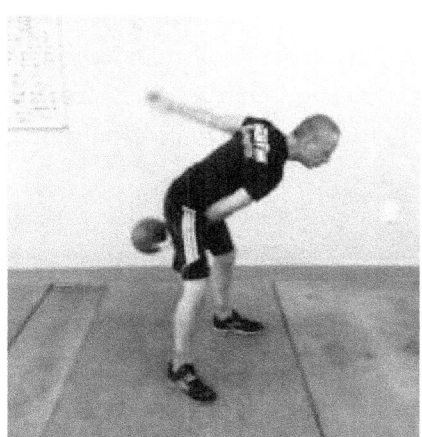

The Swing could be described as the engine that drives the kettlebell in many other lifts featured in *High Intensity Kettlebell Fitness Program*, and it's where every new lifter starts out. In Swing, the kettlebell literally swings back and forth between the lifter's legs as it's held in one hand (all lifts in the HIKF program are one-hand, one bell lifts). A lot of information that's contained in the guidelines on the Swing will be repeated with future movements. It is for that reason, we'll devote a lot of time to this deceptively technical lift. It's imperative that you master Swing, the foundation of all other lifts.

## FIRST THINGS FIRST

If you're not sure what weight bell to use, choose the lighter option. Stand about two feet behind the selected kettlebell with your feet approximately hip width apart. If you're having a hard time finding your *most balanced stance*, simply jump in place a few inches off the floor. Take note of where your feet land. Chances are this position is your most *stable platform* and the stance from which you should start. This probably will be your stance for all future lifts.

Set the angle of the bell *handle at 30 to 45 degrees* (as you look down at the floor) with the inside edge of the handle rearward. This angle allows more stability as the bell travels in a horizontal arc rearward. Keeping your feet planted, bend at the hips and place one hand over the bell handle palm down (off center towards the body's midline). Grip the handle and allow the thumb to clamp down over the index finger, forming a *finger-lock grip with the thumb over the index finger.* This mechanical lock of thumb over index finger provides additional grip strength, sparing the ring, and middle fingers (connected to finger flexors in forearm) from the having to do all the work, *preventing forearm fatigue.*

The feet are flat on the floor. The bell handle is at 45 degrees. One hand grips the bell, palm down with a finger-lock grip. The upper body is hinged over the hips with a slight knee bend forming your initial *3-Point Stance.*

## MOVING THE KETTLEBELL

Maintain a relaxed grip on the kettlebell, with the finger-lock grip engaged as you stand up. If you don't interfere with the process, the free falling bell will naturally swing back, *unless you stop it!* Be prepared, there's a good chance your arm and shoulder muscles will interfere and try and control the ascent or descent of the kettlebell on the first few swings. To help resist this urge, visualize your arm as a dangling chain, with your hand as a hook holding the kettlebell, similar to the mechanism of a wrecking ball.

*Exhale* as you *hinge at the hips* and let gravity take the bell back between your legs as far as it will go.  After the kettlebell swings all the way back, change direction, allowing the bell to swing forward. There's a definite *sweet spot* (in the direction change) that maximizes the momentum (think about being on a backyard swing), not wasting any energy as you thrust forward. If you move forward too soon, you'll miss the sweet spot and waste energy, and you'll fall short. As the bell swings back, the same angle of the bell handle is maintained, and the bell is held steady, not allowed to shake or rotate from side to side. The finger-lock grip is maintained throughout the Swing.

The arm and torso travels perfectly in time with the kettlebell, as you allow the hips to fold and the knees to unlock and go soft (this is not a deep knee bend). Much like a forward bend in yoga (with a soft knee), the back and spine are allowed to achieve a neutral position as you *follow the kettlebell.*

After the natural momentum takes the kettlebell as far back as it will go, there will be a natural direction change (bell now swinging forward), and the lifter inhales and gets the hips (glutes and hamstrings) and knees (quads) behind this forward motion at the perfect moment (earlier mentioned sweet spot). As the bell swings forward the lifters does a *slight but powerful bending and straightening of the knee joint.* The quick execution of knee bending (flexion) and straightening (extension) happens just as the bell begins to swing forward. This deliberate action actually alters the direction of the kettlebell in the forward swing, but only if the lifter's *elbow is allowed to bend* just as the knees straighten, adding a little vertical rise to an otherwise purely horizontal arc (see video). Once the knees are straightened there is no more deliberate force exerted on the kettlebell by the lifter. The forward momentum is enough to drive the bell to about waist to chest height (not higher). In this regard, the lifter is literally *riding* the bell up and down after the initial thrust forward.

As the kettlebell reaches the height of its forward motion, be sure to stand up fully and allow the back to relax. This allows the spine to achieve a neutral gravity position (skeleton is stacked), even for a brief moment, and rest (relieving back tension) before the bell changes direction and quickly drops. This seemingly weightless moment (before the bell drops) is where some of the pressure in the hand is also released and the kettlebell appears to float in front of you. You'll know you've executed a proper Swing when this *weightless moment* is first experienced.

When performed correctly, the kettlebell will drop rapidly and the lifter will need to exhale and quickly follow the bell (bend forward from the hips) while keeping the hand, torso, and kettlebell moving as one. There should be no pull or noticeable tug on arm or shoulder when the change of direction is made either on high or low part of the Swing, as the hand assumes control of the bell (fingerlock) once again. But that's possible only if the kettlebell and the body are moving in perfect sync. After a few swings, say five or ten on each side, start to notice how your *bodyweight* shifts on your feet. As the bell swings behind your body there should be a shift of bodyweight to the balls of the feet. As the bell swings forward, you should feel a shift of your body weight to the heels. When done properly, you'll get the sensation of almost scooping under the kettlebell with your hips, really feeling the work in the hips, quads, glutes, and hamstrings.

*MAIN FOCUS: The Swing is a major full body pull that works the legs, posterior chain, core, grip, and breath. When properly executed the Swing demands full use of the legs, back, core, grip, and posterior chain. It can be used as both a light warm up and heavy finisher.*

**SWING REVIEW OF MAJOR POINTS**

1. Stance
    a. 3 point stance
    b. Feet hip width or slightly wider / Jump test
2. Breathing
    a. Exhale down, inhale up
3. Finger Lock
    a. Thumb over index finger
4. Handle Angle
    a. 30 to 45 degrees
5. Force Generation
    a. Momentum
    b. Knee Extension
    c. Weight Shift
6. Follow the Kettlebell
7. Weightless Moment
8. Bent Elbow
9. Common Errors
    a. Excessive Knee Flexion
    b. Over Gripping
    c. Short Swinging
    d. Using too much upper body

## 2: CLEAN / RACK

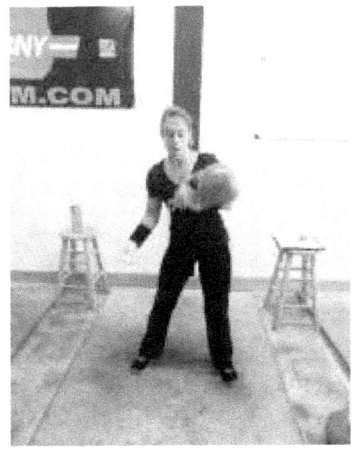

The Clean logically follows Swing in the instruction process, and involves moving the bell in one motion from the swinging motion between the legs (as in Swing) to the Rack position (chest height), where the kettlebell is briefly immobilized. The force generation is identical to the Swing, with the legs and back doing the lion's share of the work. However, clean is the first lift where the horizontal arc of the swinging kettlebell is converted to a full vertical rise. After the kettlebell is cleaned, the lifter exhales as the bell falls from Rack, swinging back between the legs, and the quickly inhales as the bell is swung back to about chest height – with another quick exhalation as the bell lands. The force behind Clean is generated with momentum (inertia of the kettlebell), the legs, back, and shifting of the body weight, really getting the hips and quads behind the movement. After the backward swing, the bell changes direction and the lifter inhales to a stand up position (Rack). The kettlebell landing is absorbed by the body, and even though we come to a hip forward position, the hip joints locks *smoothly*. This will still engage the abdominal and gluteal muscles (stabilizing the pelvis), while effectively stretching the hip flexors, keeping the low back relaxed and relatively unloaded.

In Clean, it is necessary that the lifter take advantage of the *weightless moment* (mentioned above in Swing) as the bell seems to float before it drops. This will allow the lifter to reposition their hand into the kettlebell handle with as little friction (to the palm) as possible, involving a sort of flip, where the bell *flips over the top of the hand* and lands on the hip of the palm (heel of hand pinky side), arm, chest and shoulder, directly slipping into a restful Rack position. One of the major differences between the Swing and Clean is the elbow. In Clean the elbow is kept close to the hip throughout the movement. When learning the Clean, you must, of necessity, learn the rest position of Rack.

## ONE ARM RACK POSITION

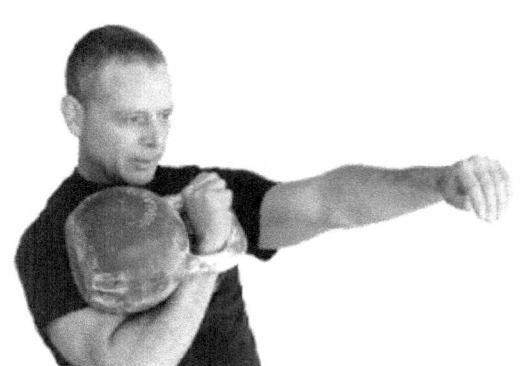

The Rack Position and Clean go hand in hand, as the Rack is the landing mat for the Clean. Once the new lifter gains confidence in either, progress follows. Each lifter will be a bit different. You may have to get the new lifter more comfortable in Rack before a decent Clean can be performed. Each case is based on many factors such as size, strength, coordination, etc. Have patience, work light, and build lifter confidence by correcting mistakes, as well as acknowledging even the most minor improvements. As the lifter develops greater flexibility, the Rack position becomes less difficult to achieve, as well as more productive (providing greater rest and a more efficient launch for Push Press and Jerk).

*The Rack Position features 4 major points:*

1. Hips are projected forward with knees straight

2. Elbow rests on the hip (if possible) with the hand rotated away from the chest

3. Bell handles lies diagonally across the palm with most of the weight on the hip of the palm

4. Wrist remains relaxed with fingers tucked behind the handle

The Rack position is unique in that it's a static position, or pause, and a opportunity for the lifter to achieve rest within the set. The lifter to uses the bone structure and connective tissue to help stabilize the kettlebell and rest between repetitions. It provides a healthy stretch of the hip flexors allowing the low back to relax, while simultaneously engaging the abdominals and gluteal muscle groups. The new lifter becomes aware of the hips (pelvis), and strength and power that lie there in. This is a win, win situation for most Americans who spend too much time seated, losing kinesthetic awareness, developing tight hips and low backs, as well as weak abs and glutes. The Rack position, as part of the Clean and LongCycle, goes a long way toward correcting this inherent problem in our modern day world.

*MAIN FOCUS: The Clean is a major full body pull that also works the legs, posterior chain, core, grip, and breath, while teaching the lifter to achieve rest between reps in the Rack position. The Rack is a powerful static stretch of the hip flexors and gentle stretch of the low back, while it develops the core and glutes.*

**REVIEW OF MAJOR POINTS**

1.  All Points Associated with Swing

    a.  Stance

    b.  Breathing (exhale down, inhale up, exhale upon landing)

    c.  Finger Lock

    d.  Handle Angle

    e.  Follow the Kettlebell

    f.  Force Generation

    g.  Elbow Stays Near Hip (in contrast to Swing)

2.  Primary Points of the Rack Position

    a.  Hips Forward with Knees Straight

    b.  Elbow on Hip (within individual's range of motion)

    c.  Wrist Relaxed (fingers tucked behind bell handle)

    d.  Bell Handle Diagonal Across Hand, on Hip of the Palm (heel of hand pinky side)

3.  Common Errors

    a.  Over Muscling (not using legs)

    b.  Inability to Achieve Rest

    c.  Wide Elbow

## 3: PRESS / LOCKOUT

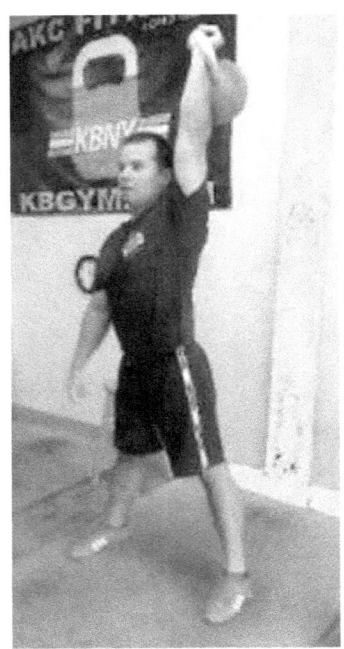

The Press requires the lifter to inhale as they push (or press) the kettlebell from Rack (chest/shoulder height) to overhead Lockout position (in a straight line up) and then exhale and literally *drop* the bell to Rack, WITHOUT the use of the legs or hips to assist in lifting the kettlebell. If necessary and pace permitting, the lifter can take one or more breathes while resting in Lockout. The Press is the first lift that requires the lifter to *fixate* the kettlebell in the overhead Lockout position. The Press is also unique in that it uses the Rack position for rest, but not as a means to *launch* (explosive use of the legs) the kettlebell to Lockout. Once locked out and fixated (no movement), the kettlebell is efficiently DROPPED, not lowered back to Rack, with no braking action (eccentric contraction) of the muscles of the shoulders and arms, but rather the force of the falling kettlebell is *absorbed* by the body (think catching a medicine ball).

*MAIN FOCUS: The Press is a high tension lift that works the major muscles of the upper body and core.*

LOCKOUT

The goal of a good Lockout is to complete the rep and to find rest. In Lockout the Kettlebell sits in the hand exactly as it does in the Rack position (handle diagonal, wrist relaxed, fingers tucked, pressure on the hip of the palm, pinky side of the hand). Improper position of the bell, as well as lack of flexibility and /or stability in the shoulder joint will greatly impact the ability stabilize the kettlebell and achieve active rest. With proper progression, practice, and patience, most lifters will gain proficiency in Lockout.

**REVIEW OF MAJOR POINTS**

1. Stance

2. Press

    a. Drop from Lockout

    b. Breathing

3. All Points Associated with Rack (see above)

4. Lockout

    a. Rest in Lockout / Fixation

    b. Relaxed Wrist / Hand

    c. Bell Handle on Hip of the Palm

    d. Elbow Locked

5. Common Errors

    a. Lack of Fixation

    b. Inability to Achieve Rest in Rack or Lockout

    c. Lowering Versus Dropping from Lockout to Rack

## SPECIAL NOTE ON FIXATION

The Press is where the new lifter will be introduced to the overhead Lockout position and the concept of fixation. The kettlebell must to come a full stop (even if briefly). Like the Rack position, Lockout is a place of rest, and also a chance for the lifter to isometrically develop the smaller stabilizer muscles of the shoulder joint, protecting the shoulder from future injury, building strength, flexibility, and stability.

## 4: PUSH PRESS

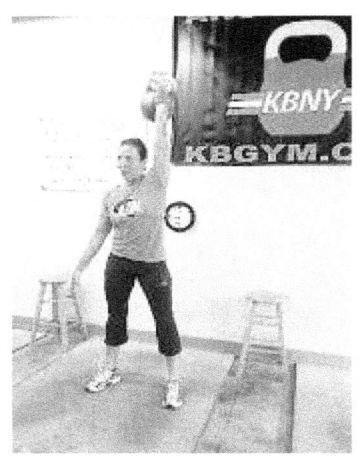

Once the basics of Press are learned, the Push Press is the next logical step. The Push Press is similar to Press, but incorporates a single knee dip (from the knees not hips) and the use of the legs to help propel the kettlebell from Rack to Lockout (finishing the lift with the arm and shoulder). The breathing pattern is the same as Press, as you inhale as the bell travels up, exhale as it drops down. The Push Press is the first explosive push exercise that incorporates the larger, more powerful muscles of the lower body to launch the kettlebell to Lockout. During Push Press, the heels remain on flat on the floor (no ankle or foot involvement).

*MAIN FOCUS: The Push Press is a full body exercise that teaches, as well as motivates, the lifter to use their entire body (upper, lower, core) as one efficient unit to repeatedly generate maximum force.*

**REVIEW OF MAJOR POINTS**

1. Stance

2. Rack Reviewed

3. Single Dip

4. Powerful Heave (Launch)

   a. Feet remain planted on floor

5. Lockout Reviewed

6. Drop Reviewed

7. Breathing

8. Common Errors

   a. Lack of Fixation

   b. Inadequate Dip / Use of Legs

   c. Over Muscling

   d. Inability to Achieve Rest in Rack or Lockout

   e. Lowering Versus Dropping from Lockout to Rack

## 5: JERK

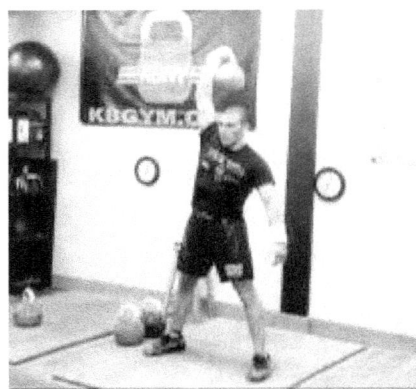

The Jerk builds on Push Press and adds a quick second dip (known as the *double-dip*). In other words, after the bell is launched from the hip (inhale), there is an immediate change of direction (of the body, not the kettlebell) as the lifter drops under the rising kettlbell to achieve overhead Lockout (elbow locks). The knees are then straightened to complete the rep. The lifter can breathe in Lockout if necessary, but the bell is then dropped back to the Rack position as the lifter exhales (as in Press and Push Press). The double-dip of the Jerk can be initially difficult to master and there should be no rush to include the more advanced movements of Jerk and Snatch until comfortable with the Press, Push Press, Swing and Clean.

 In Jerk, the lifter comes up on his or her toes, bringing into play the explosive calf muscles (ankle flexion) as well as the powerful hips and knees. The ankle-foot action provides a concentrated explosive pop from the calf muscles. The new lifter needs to develop flexibility in the ankle joint, as well as learn to coordinate the ankles, knees, and hips, in a powerfully explosive launch of the kettlebell, via a direct elbow hip connection, before full potential is realized.

*MAIN FOCUS: The Jerk not only works the major muscles of the upper and lower body, as well as core, but develops explosive power, timing, and speed.*

**REVIEW OF MAJOR POINTS**

1. Stance

2. Rack Reviewed

3. Single Dip

4. Explosive Pop (Launch)

    a. Lifter come up on toes (engaging explosive calf muscle)

5. Double Dip

6. Lockout Reviewed

7. Drop Reviewed)

8. Breathing

9. Common Errors

    a. Lack of Fixation

    b. Inadequate First Dip / Use of Legs

    c. Lack of Double Dip

    d. Over Muscling

    e. Inability to Achieve Rest in Rack or Lockout

    f. Lowering Versus Dropping from Lockout to Rack

# 6: LONGCYCLE / VARIATIONS

**VIDEO: CLICK HERE**

DOWNLOAD: CLICK HERE

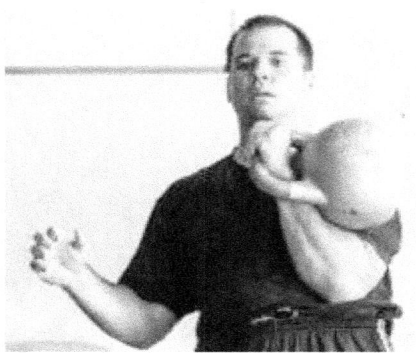

The LongCycle includes three variations, but always involves lifting the kettlebell in two phases. First the bell is Cleaned to the Rack position (see section on Clean above), then either Pressed (see P12 on Press), Push Pressed (see P13 on Push Press), or Jerked (see P14 on Jerk) to overhead Lockout. The LongCycle is the ultimate, single-set, full body workout.

*MAIN FOCUS: The LongCycle combines pulling and pushing power, to give the lifter an extremely efficient full body workout, working*

## REVIEW OF MAJOR POINTS

1. Stance
2. Clean and Jerk
3. Rack Reviewed
4. Single Dip
5. Launch
6. Double Dip
7. Lockout Reviewed
8. Breathing
9. Drop Reviewed
10. Common Errors
    a. Lack of Fixation
    b. Excessive Hip Flexion

## 7: HALF SNATCH

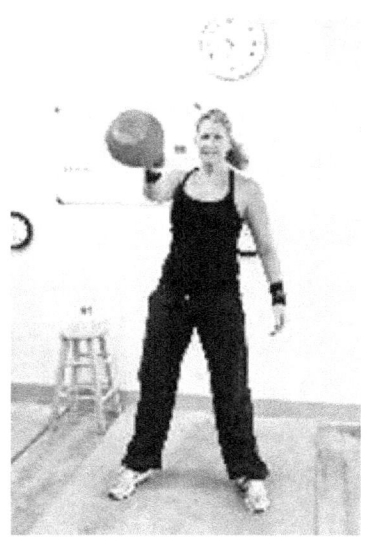

The Half Snatch takes the kettlebell from a position swinging between the legs, directly to overhead Lockout, in one fluid motion. The lifter inhales as the bell is pulled (much like Swing) from between the legs directly to Lockout. The lifter exhales as the kettlebell is dropped to Rack. The lifter can find rest in both Rack and Lockout (being sure to breathe). The lifter exhales and drops the bell from Rack as in a Clean), and the kettlebell is re-Snatched to lockout with a big inhalation on the way up. The Half Snatch (and Snatch) requires the lifter to be aggressive. Insufficient aggression will show up as lack of fluidity and speed, and will not allow the bell to move at its true force and efficiency. The lifter ends up with bad timing, forced to muscle the kettlebell to achieve Lockout. This will eventually result in an overuse injury. It's important to understand the necessity to come out of the extreme rearward bend (following the kettlebell) with an appropriate level of aggression, engaging the legs and back. Don't think of Snatching just as an upper body or arm exercise. Use the force generators learned in Swing to get the bell to the overhead Lockout position.

DROP FROM RACK

After the bell is dropped from the Rack position, the lifter follows the kettlebell, with the head and torso, between the legs, and gets ready for an immediate change in direction (inhaling) and re-snatches the kettlebell. The lifter needs to *feel* when the bell finishes its rearward swing. It is at this crucial moment they must aggressively change direction and move forward, while rising to a stand up position propelling the kettlebell to Lockout. The bell and lifter's hand (hip of the palm) should meet up in the Lockout position, arriving at the exact same moment, making for a smooth landing. All the work is done at the initial pull.

For some the Half Snatch, as well as Snatch, can be difficult to master. We have found that allowing a new lifter to perform a few Swings in conjunction with Half Snatch eases the learning process. A suggested sequence would be repeating the pattern of three Swings followed by one Half Snatch. As the lifter gains confidence and proficiency, they can eliminate the Swing entirely from rep sequence.

*MAIN FOCUS: The Half Snatch develops pulling power and works the posterior chain, legs, core, grip and breath.*

## REVIEW OF MAJOR POINTS

1. Stance

2. Fingerlock Reviewed

3. Handle Angle

4. Snatch (pull force generation)

    a. Timing

    b. Momentum

    c. Legs and Posterior Chain

5. Lockout Reviewed

6. Drop to Rack

7. Breathing (1)

8. Common Errors

    a. Poor timing

    b. Lack of fingerlock

    c. Improper handle angle

    d. Improper swing depth

    e. Overbending of the knees

    f. Lack of fixation

## 8: SNATCH

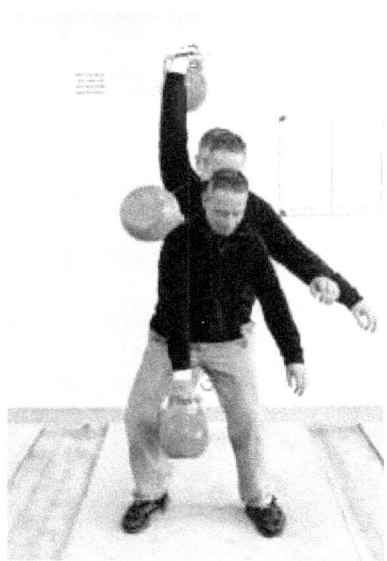

Like Half Snatch, the full version of Snatch takes the bell from a position between the legs to overhead Lockout in one move, but then drops the bell from Lockout to back between the legs (bypassing the Rack position). The kettlebell is then immediately re-snatched directly to Lockout. The Snatch (and Half Snatch) requires the lifter to be aggressive. Insufficient aggression will show up as lack of fluidity and speed, will not allow the bell to achieve maximum force and efficiency. The lifter ends up with bad timing, while resorting to muscling (using too much arm) the kettlebell. This will result in an eventual overuse injury. It's important to come out of the extreme rearward position (following the kettlebell) aggressively, engaging the legs and back. Don't think of Snatching as just an upper body or arm exercise. Use the force generators learned in Swing to allow the bell to float up the front your body and land on a dime (on the hip of the palm), in the identical lockout position of Press, Push Press, and Jerk.

DROP FROM LOCKOUT

The drop from overhead Lockout (versus to Rack) is one of the last major skills a new lifter needs to learn. Typically, he or she will have mastered the other skills associated with advanced Snatch and Jerk, and will have developed a strong Lockout. As the bell sits in Lockout, perched on the hip of the palm, it's in a position to easily leave the hand (drop) and cascade down the front of the body. This is accomplished by a simple rotation (turn thumb to rear) of the arm and hand toward the midline of the body (exhaling). The bell will appear to free fall, as the lifter rides the kettlebell down to its lowest, most rearward position, *following* the kettlebell between the legs (see instruction on Swing and Clean). It's important to remember that the arm collapses (elbow bends) only after the bell has actually left the hand and begins its descent. The lifter then follows the kettlebell with the head and torso, between the legs. After the bell has finished its rearward arc, there is an immediate change direction (inhale) as the lifter immediately and aggressively re-snatches another rep. The lifter needs to *feel* when the bell finishes its rearward swing. It is at this crucial moment that he must aggressively change direction, get the quads into the act, and move forward (inhaling), while rising to a fully standing position with the bell landing easily in Lockout. The bell and lifter's hand (hip of the palm) should meet up in the Lockout position, arriving at the *exact* same moment, making for a smooth landing, and a smooth rep.

*MAIN FOCUS: The Snatch is a full body lift, with focus on extreme pulling power, overall conditioning, posterior chain, legs, core, grip and breath.*

**REVIEW OF MAJOR POINTS**

1. Stance
2. Fingerlock Reviewed (1)
3. Snatch (pull force generation)
    a. Timing
    b. Momentum
    c. Legs and Poster Chain
4. Snatch Drop
    a. Importance of proper lockout
    b. Letting the bell fall
    c. Following the bell
5. Breathing
6. Common Errors
    a. Poor Timing
    b. Lack of Fingerlock
    c. Improper handle angle
    d. Improper swing depth
    e. Over bending of the knees
    f. Lack of fixation
    g. Improper drop
    h. Holding the Breath

## CHALK APPLICATION

Chalk is an important aspect of kettlebell lifting, especially for kettlebell sport lifts, but chalk also plays a major role in the HIKF program. Chalk, when properly applied, on both the kettlebell handle and the lifter's hands, provides the perfect level of friction to not limit the set, while keeping hands healthy. Moisture is the enemy that will end a set long before the larger muscles of the legs, back are done, or the heart and lungs are sufficiently challenged. The use of chalk, combined with proper technique will make a huge difference in exercises that require a major pull (where grip strength-endurance is involved), such as Swing, Clean, Half Snatch and especially Snatch. The goal of a well chalked kettlebell is not to have excess chalk rain down from the kettlebell during the lift. The chalk should be rubbed deeply into the handle (and the hands), and "stick" to the metal surface. Sometimes this can take some time and patience, and very small amount of moisture (from a water spray bottle) can be applied to the handle, but only if absolutely necessary to get the chalk to adhere or speed up the process. Avoid using too much water, less is more.

BONUS CHALK VIDEO: CLICK HERE

# III: THE 7 VARIABLES

*This section introduces the Seven Variables and breaks down each one. The lifter gains insight on how to integrate the variables so as to control the intensity and overall effect of the exercise session. The same set can be dramatically altered with a simple change of a single variable.*

## 1: LIFT SELECTION

First and foremost, kettlebell lift selection sets the intention, tone and intensity level of the workout, and defines the workout session. The 8 Core Kettlebell Fitness Lifts can be performed *singularly* (one lift encompasses the entire sequence), or in combination (a series of different lifts make up the workout) based on the specific PROTOCOL being followed (for 15 pre-established PROTOCOLs that incorporate multiple exercises performed in a specific sequence, see Part III).  As found in the technique section of this manual, the following 8 lifts are at the kettlebell lifter or trainer's disposal, for use with the 15 pre-established PROTOCOLs as well as in generating their own routines.

**THE 8 LIFTS**

1.  SWING
    a.  Full body with emphasis on legs, grip, breath, posterior chain
2.  CLEAN
    a.  Full body, with emphasis on legs, grip, arms, posterior chain
3.  PRESS
    a.  Upper body, with emphasis on arms, shoulders
4.  PUSH PRESS
    a.  Full body, with emphasis on legs, arms, shoulders
5.  JERK
    a.  Full body with emphasis on explosive power, legs
6.  LONGCYCLE (variations)
    a.  Full body with emphasis on legs, as well as the push and pull aspects of lifting
7.  HALF SNATCH
    a.  Full body with emphasis on legs, posterior chain, breath
8.  SNATCH

    a.   Full body with emphasis on legs, posterior chain, grip, breath

Exercise selection is limited by the lifter's proficiency level with each move. Until a minimum level of skill is reached, new lifters are restricted to exercises where proficiency is adequate and a safety is assured. There is no set timetable for this process, as each lifter will develop at his, or her, own pace. Attention to detail, practice, and patience will be required by the lifter and instructor to ensure new lifters develop as rapidly, yet as safely, as possible, with each succeeding workout building a more solid foundation for an increased workload and greater intensity levels (where results lie).

While HIKF generally demands an almost constant full body effort, each exercise selected (along with the other variables) will determine the *primary effect* of the workout (strength, endurance, weight loss, explosive power, speed, job and task specific, etc.).

## 2: SEQUENCING

All kettlebell fitness routines should reflect the goals of the lifter. Sequencing, refers to the order the movements. For single exercise routines, this variable does not apply. There is a logic behind how movements are grouped and ordered. For most multi-movement routines, there is usually a combination of push and pull in every PROTOCOL, but there are exceptions. Let's take a look at three HIFK Zero Rest PROTOCOLs (see Part III).

A 20 minute Long Cycle set performed at 1 minute per hand (Long Cycle involves a Clean combined with a Jerk, Push Press, or Press) is a 20 minute full body, push and pull workout. No muscle group is left untouched. This allows the body to perform more work as the work is distributed around the body. Another HIKF PROTOCOL, the Jerk and Half Snatch Mirror, uses the Jerk and Half Snatch in 4 minute sequences for 20 minutes. Again, a full body workout is achieved, but comes at it from a different angle, combing 4 minute segments of pushing (Jerk) with 4 minute segments of pulling (Half Snatch). Last but not least, let's look at the 16 minute Kitchen Sink. This PROTOCOL utilizes all 8 movements listed in the HIKF program. Every muscle group is involved but emphasis (exercise) switches every two minutes, allowing high intensity with very little chance of overuse or failure.

Part III presents 15 pre-established kettlebell PROTOCOLs, as well as three examples of HIKF Cross Performance routines. After you complete the program, and become proficient in proper technique, as well as learn to manipulate the seven variables, trainers and lifters are encouraged to generate their own HIKF routines. Programs should be based on realistic goals and the seven variables contained in this manual. Until you feel 100 percent confident in developing your own programs, operate within the pre-established programs presented in Part III.

## 3: KETTLEBELL SELECTION

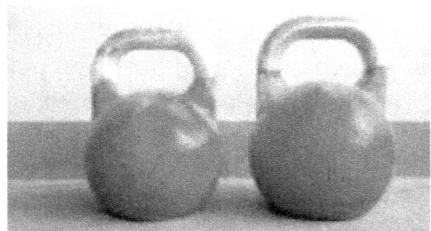

Pro Grade, or *Competition Sytle* Kettlebells were introduced in the United States in 2007 by Valery Fedorenko with the formation American Kettlebell Club®. Today, there are numerous manufactures and distributors of these competition style kettlebells, which are made of cast steel to exact dimension. Regardless of the weight of the kettlebell, Pro Grade bells are the same size and shape but come in colors that match their relative kilogram. They come in two sizes, including a newly released smaller bell more appropriate for a person of smaller stature. Bells traditionally range in weight from 8 kilograms (18 pounds) to 48 kilograms (106 pounds) at 2 kilogram increments. Even lighter bells are soon to be released. Deciding the appropriate weight kettlebell to use will be addressed in Variable 3. The World Kettlebell Club® is the original manufacturer and best source for Pro Grade, Performance, Fitness and Precision Kettlebells.

Professional Grade kettlebells are also used in competition, with strict adherence to specifications. Athletes traditionally compete in the Biathlon (Jerk and Snatch) and LongCycle with bells ranging from 12 kilograms to 32 kilograms and more. Sport training is, however, the topic of another course.

Only *Professional Grade Kettlebells* (or the like, see above) are appropriate for use with this program. Pro Grade kettlebells come in sizes from ranging from 4 kilograms to 48 kilograms and more. For the purpose of this program, most novice female lifters should start with an 8kg or 10kg, and beginner male lifters will usually start with either 12kg or 16kg. Always err on the side of caution when choosing the weight of the kettlebell. A good rule of thumb, especially for beginners, *is to lift light and lift right!* More often than not, technique is safely mastered with relatively light weight. Once this has been accomplished, it may be the right time to incorporate a heavier bell.

In sequenced sets that employ more than one lift (see Part III), kettlebell selection will be limited by the most difficult lift in the sequence. For example, the Snatch is the most technical movement (that's part of this program manual), and normally would require a lighter kettlebell than Jerk, so in a sequenced set involving both Jerk and Snatch, the kettlebell most appropriate for Snatch would have to be used (unless you incorporate a mid-stream switch). The use of all seven variables, *in combination,* are used to generate the appropriate intensity level for each set, each lifter.

## 4: SET LENGTH

Set length will vary from as short as two minutes (or less if necessary) to 20 minutes (and possibly longer). Set length, usually expressed in *minutes*, is one of the primary adjustments that assist the kettlebell lifter in achieving a specific goal (IE: weight loss, general fitness, strength, endurance, speed, power, etc.) and intensity level. During a typical kettlebell set, once the bell is picked up, it is generally not set down until the set is complete (clock runs out). Certain PROTOCOLs include more than one set (of equal or variable length), with a timed rest period between movements. The approach to rest will be addressed with Variable Number 6: *Rest Between Sets*. With sequenced sets that involve more than one kettlebell lift, consider the rest period between each movement to be zero. During the initial instruction phase, the new lifter must adjust each variable, including set length. As the he or she masters proper technique, the potential for longer sets will eventually be achieved (in most healthy individuals). While it is sometimes possible to bring the new lifter from 2 minute to 20 minute sets in a relatively short time, it is usually best to progress slowly, emphasizing technique development without cranking up the Seven Intensity Variables before technique is developed.

When first graduating to longer sets, it is also suggested that the lifter reduce the intensity of other variables, especially the weight of the kettlebell, how often the bell is transferred from hand to hand (expressed in minutes per hand or MPH), and at what pace (expressed in reps per minute or RPM) the bell is lifted. For most beginners, it is recommended to use a structured approach, following a pre-determined progression. Be flexible and adjust progression as needed, either slower or faster. In other words, it's okay to repeat or skip levels when and where appropriate, at your discretion.

## INTITIAL 12 STEP PROGRESSION*

1. 4 Minute Set
2. 6 Minute Set
3. 2, 4 Minute Sets
4. 8 Minute Set

5. 2, 6 Minute Sets

6. 10 Minute Set

7. 12 Minute Set

8. 2, 8 Minute Sets

9. 16 Minute Set

10. 18 Minute Set

11. 2, 10 Minute Sets

12. 20 Minute Set

*Trainers and athletes are advised to use the 12 step progression as a general guide only. Adjust set length to the capacity of the individual at their current level. Repeat or skip levels when and where appropriate. A single lift, or a combination of movements, may be utilized.*

## 5: MINUTES PER HAND (MPH)

It's easy to see that varying how often the kettlebell is switched from hand to hand will have a dramatic impact on the overall intensity of the set. The concept of a single hand switch in a ten minute set is what defines many kettlebell sport sets, which is *not* the topic of this manual. However, there is tremendous benefit to be gained by controlling how long the kettlebell will be lifted per hand. At the surface, it seems fairly logical that allowing frequent hand switches will transfer much of the intensity from the upper body to the legs, core, and breath, but this not always the case.

When the upper body reaches *nearly complete fatigue,* the legs are heavily motivated to go into action. With an experienced lifter, you'll notice that every rep looks the same, the legs working at full capacity from rep one. It is for this reason that some single switch sets need to be incorporated early on – as wake up call to the lower body. While the five minute per hand, ten minute set option isn't absolutely necessary to master technique (unless you're a competitive Kettlebell Sport athlete), this methodology should be in the tool box of every Kettlebell Fitness trainer and lifter. Taking a lifter to two minutes per hand on a regular basis (at least weekly) and three minutes per hand occasionally (at least monthly) within their regular workouts is an important aspect of learning to tap into the power of the hips, back, and legs, as well as motivating the lifter to find rest in the Rack and Lockout positions.

With many of the pre-established, time-tested PROTOCOLs found in Part III: Exercise Combinations and Routines, sequenced sets with or without rest can be intensified by increasing hand switches beyond one minute per hand to two, three, and on occasion, four and five minutes per hand (this applies to the high level, and well-motivated athlete).

Remember, this variable can have a tremendous impact on any set, but sometimes its benefit is hard to appreciate. In the short run, performing one switch sets may reduce overall set length, and therefore reduce the workload on the core and lower body, but this process facilitates long term activation of the larger muscles of legs, hips, and core by instinctively encouraging the lifter to use their legs.

## 6: REPS PER MINUTE (RPM)

We all understand the concept of pace in activities like running, but with High Intensity Kettlebell Fitness, controlling pace may be the hardest variable for the new lifter to master. Depending upon lifter goals or PROTOCOL design, sometimes a rapid pace is called for. However, at the very early stages of the cognitive learning process, a slower pace is usually preferred, mainly to assist in technique assimilation. Once technique is mastered, controlling reps performed each minute (RPM), maintaining a relatively even pace (whether slow, medium or fast), is a powerful tool that gives the lifter precision control over the intensity of any set.

Speed (high rep per minute ranges) can be as effective an intensity booster as an increase in resistance (weight of kettlebell).  But buyer beware, speed can also ruin technique, especially at the early stages – opening a new lifter to needless injury.  Be sure every new lifter masters proper form before working at the highest rep ranges.

Below is a list of general rep ranges. Some of the progressions and PROTOCOLs listed in the next section will come with specific rep per minute guidelines. Remember not all lifters are created equal, when it comes to technique and capacity. Adjust for the individual.

## REP RANGE CHART

*Expressed in reps per minute / RPM*

1. **SWING**: 30 to 35 RPM (no control here)*

2. **CLEAN**: 6 to 20 RPM

3. **PRESS**: 6 to 12 RPM

4. **PUSH PRESS**: 6 to 20 RPM

5. **JERK**: 6 to 20 RPM

6. **LONGCYCLE**: 4 to 12 RPM

7. **HALF SNATCH**: 6 to 18 RPM

8. **SNATCH**: 12 to 20 RPM

*The swing varies from other lifts in that the lifter has no real control over the pace. Most lifters will work at somewhere between 30 and 35 reps per minute (RPM)

## 7: REST BETWEEN SETS

By manipulating the rest taken between each set, the lifter can dramatically alter the overall intensity of any workout. Rest can vary from zero (the lifter moves directly from one exercise to the next in the same set without stopping) to as long as five minutes or more (allowing recovery time between sets). Higher end rest (above 3 minutes) applies mainly to kettlebell sport training, where *full* rest is required to perform at your best. Many of our HIKF pre-established PROTOCOLs (presented in Part III), will utilize a 1 to 3 minute recovery period. This allows the lifter to potentially work harder overall.

When creating Cross Performance programs (integrating kettlebell movements with other non-kettlebell exercises), the time between sets may be filled with another exercise. For example:

*SAMPLE HIKF CROSS PERFORMANCE ROUTINE WITH ACTIVE REST BETWEEN SETS*

1.  Jerk: 4 minutes at 2 minutes per hand followed by 20 bodyweight squats
2.  Snatch:4 minutes at 2 minutes per hand followed by 10 pull ups
3.  LongCycle: 4 minutes at 2 minutes per hand followed by 10 minutes of rowing

There are three Cross Performance routines, six *Zero Rest* kettlebell routines, and *six Recovery* routines presented in Part III

## SPECIAL NOTE ON FREQUENCY

Kettlebell lifting, is unique as a resistance exercise modality, because the same movements, albeit worked at various intensity levels, can be repeated daily.  It's up to the new lifter to find a formula that works based on the *intensity duration formula arrived at each workout, as well as the lifter's personal attributes (IE: resiliency and work capacity),* to determine optimum frequency of your  training. This can sometimes be a complicated formula to arrive at, as there are no strict limitations on how often someone can train, other than at least one rest day per week is essential (even at the highest level). As a rule of thumb, three or four HIKF workouts per week is a good place to start. This gives the lifter a chance to better gauge (based on the above formula) his or her work capacity, or when training becomes overtraining. At the highest level, five or six days per week are recommended.

## 7 VARIABLES IN REVIEW

1. LIFT SELECTION
2. KETTLEBELL SELECTION
3. SET LENGTH
4. MINUTES PER HAND (mph)
5. REPS PER MINUTE (rpm)
6. SEQUENCING
7. REST BETWEEN SETS

# IV: HIKF ROUTINES AND PROTOCOLS

*In this section we will expand upon Initial 12-Step Progression, introduce 6 Zero Rest Routines, 6Recovery Routines, and three examples of Cross Performance Routines that make up the HIKF PROTOCOLs.*

It is highly recommended that the new lifter follow an initial progression the builds the necessary level of technique, stability, and mobility before progressing to more intense training. However, High Intensity Kettlebell Fitness can rapidly reach extreme levels, with an enormous cardiovascular demand.

HIKF training can place a high demand on the cardiovascular system. Get clearance from your physician before beginning. Utilize this Initial 12-Step Progress (below), to gradually increase your work capacity.

## INTITIAL SUGGESTED 12 STEP PROGRESSION

All sets are at performed at 1 to 2 minutes per hand*

1. 4 Minute Set

2. 6 Minute Set

3. 2, 4 Minute Sets

4. 8 Minute Set

5. 2, 6 Minute Sets

6. 10 Minute Set

7. 12 Minute Set

8. 2, 8 Minute Sets

9. 16 Minute Set

10. 18 Minute Set

11. 2, 10 Minute Sets

12. 20 Minute Set

New trainers and lifters are advised to follow the 12 step progression, using the above sequence as a general guide. Adjust set length to the capacity of the individual at their current level. The lifter should repeat or skip levels when and where appropriate. One exercise, or a combination of lifts, may be utilized, depending upon the lifter's proficiency with each lift during the initial learning process. New lifts many be introduced while working through the progression. Remember, besides building the physical capacity to handle regular extended or multiple sets, the new lifter must also psychologically acclimate, developing the mind-set and mental fortitude necessary to complete a nonstop 20-minute, high intensity workout. Time, patience, determinate, dedication, and technique mastery is an absolute must if the lifter is to be successful, and remain healthy.

# HIKF ZERO REST PROTOCOL©

## 1: POLICE PROTOCOL

*The Chase and Grapple*

1. **KETTLEBELL KG**: Variable

2. **TOTAL SET LENGTH**: 8 Minutes

3. **MIN PER EXERCISE**: 4 Minutes

4. **SWITCH / MPH:** 1 or 2

5. **PACE /RPM GOALS**: See RPM Chart  / Jerk fast, Clean slow

6. **EXERCISE SEQUENCE**: Perform Jerk at 4 minutes light and at a faster pace, followed by Clean for 4 minutes, heavier (switch bells quickly) and at a slower pace.

HOW THIS WORKOUT DEVELOPED

At Gym KBNY, we have a lot of law enforcement workers, such as cops, court and correction officers, who are called upon to chase down, then grapple with a potential criminal. This workout was designed to assist with that.

# HIKF ZERO REST PROTOCOL©

## 2: 10 MINUTE PENTATHLON

*The Mini-Q*

1. **KETTLEBELL KG**: Variable

2. **TOTAL SET LENGTH**: 10 Minutes

3. **MIN PER EXERCISE**: 2 Minutes

4. **SWITCH / MPH:** 1

5. **PACE /RPM GOALS**: See RPM Chart / work at a moderate to fast pace

6. **EXERCISE SEQUENCE**: Perform 2 minutes of Clean, followed by 2 minutes of LongCycle Press, followed by 2 minutes of Jerk, followed by 2 minutes of Half Snatch, followed by 2 minutes of Push Press.

HOW THIS WORKOUT DEVELOPED

A version of the Kettlebell Pentathlon performed in one 10 minute set makes the perfect "mini" workout. Don't fool yourself, this one can be tough if you use the right weight, and go fast enough. .

# HIKF ZERO REST PROTOCOL©

## 3: 12 MINUTE JERK

*Jerk Slide*

1. **KETTLEBELL KG**: Variable

2. **TOTAL SET LENGTH**:12 Minutes

3. **MIN PER EXERCISE**:2 Minutes

4. **HAND SWITCHES IN MPH:** 3-2-1

5. **PACE /RPM GOALS**: See RPM Chart / work at a slower pace during the 3 mph phase, a moderate pace at the 2 mph phase, and faster pace at the 1 mph phase, of the set.

6. **EXERCISE SEQUENCE**: Perform 12 straight minutes of Jerk at 3 minutes per hand, 2 minutes per hand, and 1 mph

HOW THIS WORKOUT DEVELOPED

Don't let this one fool you. In only 12 minutes, this is one of the most intense workouts in this eBook. But it starts tough, and gets "easier" as the set progresses.

# HIKF ZERO REST PROTOCOL©

## 4: 16 MINUTES OF EVERYTHING

*The Kitchen Sink*

1. **KETTLEBELL KG**: Variable

2. **TOTAL SET LENGTH**:16 Minutes

3. **MIN PER EXERCISE**:2 Minutes

4. **HAND SWITCHES IN MPH:** 1

5. **PACE /RPM GOALS:** See RPM Chart / work from a moderate to fast pace

6. **EXERCISE SEQUENCE**: Perform 2 minutes Clean, followed by 2 minutes of LongCycle Press, followed by 2 minutes of Jerk, followed by 2 minutes of Snatch, followed by 2 minutes of Push Press, followed by 2 minutes of Half Snatch, followed by 2 minutes of LongCycle, followed by 2 minutes of Swing.

HOW THIS WORKOUT DEVELOPED

The Kitchen Sink is one of the favorite workouts at Gym KBNY, and the test I give at the end of every live trainer course. It includes all 8 core lifts, and is a great way to learn all the lifts and get an intense workout.

# HIKF ZERO REST PROTOCOL©

## 5: 16-MINUTE NEVER-QUIT

*Firefighter PROTOCOL*

1. **KETTLEBELL KG**: Variable

2. **TOTAL SET LENGTH**: 16 Minutes

3. **MIN PER EXERCISE**: 4 Minutes

4. **HAND SWITCHES IN MPH:** 1 to 4

5. **PACE /RPM GOALS**: See RPM Chart / work slow if working at 4MPH, moderate if working at 2 MPH, and fast if working at 1MPH

6. **EXERCISE SEQUENCE**: Perform 8 minutes of Push Press at 1 to 4MPH, followed by 8 minutes of Half Snatch at 1 to 4MPH

HOW THIS WORKOUT DEVELOPED

The Firefighter PROTOCOL is back to my roots and based on what a firefighter is required to do at just about every structural fire. Work for about 15 or 17 minutes (time allowed by an air pac). Most of the work is either pulling, or pushing, the two basic human movements. There is a lot of variation in this program, as you can work anywhere from 1 to 4 minutes per hand. The less you switch, the slower you go.

# HIKF ZERO REST PROTOCOL©

## 6: 20-MINUTE PURE FOCUS

*Snatch or LongCycle Marathon*

1. **KETTLEBELL KG**: Variable

2. **TOTAL SET LENGTH**: 20 Minutes

3. **MIN PER EXERCISE**: 20 Minutes

4. **HAND SWITCHES IN MPH:** 1 or 2

5. **PACE /RPM GOALS:** See RPM Chart / varies with weight use

6. **EXERCISE SEQUENCE**: Perform either LongCycle or Snatch straight through for 20 minutes. Pace will vary with proficiency, weight used, and whether you switch hands at 1 or 2 minute intervals

HOW THIS WORKOUT DEVELOPED

To be able to perform a straight 20 minute set is a badge of honor at our gym. In this old favorite, you can work with either LongCycle or Snatch, switching at 1 or 2 minutes per hand. Lots of variables here to make this a jog, sprint, or heavy set.

# HIKF RECOVERY PROTOCOL©

## 7: STRONGMAN

*Heavy Handed*

1. **KETTLEBELL KG**: Variable BUT Heavy

2. **TOTAL SETS**: 3

3. **REST BETWEEN SETS**: 2 Minutes

4. **TOTAL SET LENGTH**: All 4 Minutes

5. **HAND SWITCHES IN MPH:** 2

6. **PACE /RPM GOALS**: See RPM Chart / Jerk 12 –Clean 12 – LongCycle 12

7. **EXERCISE SEQUENCE**: Perform Jerk at 4 minutes / 2 mph / as heavy as you can handle with a rpm goal of 12 / REST 2 MINUTES – Perform Clean at 4 minutes / 2 mph / as heavy as you can handle with a rpm goal of 12 – Perform LongCycle at 4 minutes / 2 mph / as heavy as you can handle with a rpm goal of 12

HOW THIS WORKOUT DEVELOPED

Based on Kettlebell StrongSport competitions, this gives the newer lifter a chance to work strength as the main focus of his or her training. At 2 minute per hand sets, still real tough.

# HIKF RECOVERY PROTOCOL©

## 8: CONDITIONING SEQUENCE

*Kettlle Hell*

1.  **KETTLEBELL KG**: Variable

2.  **TOTAL SETS**: 3

3.  **REST BETWEEN SETS**: 1 Minute

4.  **TOTAL SET LENGTH**: All 6 Minutes

5.  **HAND SWITCHES IN MPH:** 1

6.  **PACE /RPM GOALS**: See RPM Chart / Work at the high end paces

    listed

7.  **EXERCISE SEQUENCE**: Perform Jerk at 6 minutes / 1mph fast / REST

    1 MINUTE– Perform Snatch at 6 minutes / 1mph fast / REST 1

    MINUTE– Perform LongCycle at 6 minutes / 1mph fast

HOW THIS WORKOUT DEVELOPED

A lot of high school wrestlers train at Gym KBNY, and this workout was designed to mimic the match and round sequence of six minutes on, one rest, the young wrestlers must follow. True hell with only one minute rest.

# HIKF RECOVERY PROTOCOL©

## 9: HIGH INTENSITY

*Crazy 8's*

1. **KETTLEBELL KG**: Variable

2. **TOTAL SETS**: 3

3. **REST BETWEEN SETS**: 2 to 3 Minute

4. **TOTAL SET LENGTH**: All 8 Minutes

5. **HAND SWITCHES IN MPH**: 1

6. **PACE /RPM GOALS**: See RPM Chart / Work at the moderate paces listed

7. **EXERCISE SEQUENCE**: Perform Jerk at 8 minutes / 1mph / REST 1 MINUTE– Perform Snatch at 8 minutes / 1mph / REST 1 MINUTE– Perform LongCycle at 8 minutes / 1mph

HOW THIS WORKOUT DEVELOPED

Beside the great name, it takes Kettle Hell to a whole new level, and your total set time is 24 minutes. Super high intensity here.

# HIKF RECOVERY PROTOCOL©

## 10: SET REDUCTION

*The Time Machine*

1. **KETTLEBELL KG**: Variable

2. **TOTAL SETS**: 3

3. **REST BETWEEN SETS**: 2 Minutes

4. **TOTAL SET LENGTH**: 12 Minutes, 8 Minutes, and 4 Minutes

5. **HAND SWITCHES IN MPH:** 1 to 2 mph

6. **PACE /RPM GOALS**: See RPM Chart / work at slow, moderate, and fast pace

7. **EXERCISE SEQUENCE**: Select from any of the 8 core exercises. Stick with the same exercise through the entire sequence. The first set is done at 12 minutes / 1 to 2 mph. working at a slow pace. The second set is done at 8 minutes / 1 to 2 minutes per hand, working at a moderate pace. The last set is done at 4 minutes / 1 to 2 minutes per hand, working at a fast pace. Rest 2 minutes between all sets.

HOW THIS WORKOUT DEVELOPED

The idea behind this set is to trick the body into performing more efficiently in longer sets, by manipulating speed and hand switches in the same set. Works like a charm.

# HIKF RECOVERY PROTOCOL©

## 11: FIVE-PACK

*4 X 5*

1. **KETTLEBELL KG**: Variable

2. **TOTAL SETS**: 5

3. **REST BETWEEN SETS**: 2 Minutes

4. **TOTAL SET LENGTH**: All 4 Minutes

5. **HAND SWITCHES IN MPH:** 1 mph

6. **PACE /RPM GOALS**: See RPM Chart / fast pace

7. **EXERCISE SEQUENCE**: Perform the Clean at 4 minutes / 1 mph / 2 minutes rest – : Perform the LongCycle Press at 4 minutes / 1 mph / 2 minutes rest –: Perform the Jerk at 4 minutes / 1 mph / 2 minutes rest –: Perform the Half Snatch at 4 minutes / 1 mph / 2 minutes rest –: Perform the Push Press at 4 minutes / 1 mph

HOW THIS WORKOUT DEVELOPED

Five sets, four minutes each, 2 minutes rest, fast pace suggested. You do the math. This sequence is one tough mother.

# HIKF RECOVERY PROTOCOL©

## 12: VARIED INTENSITY

*Pyramid Power*

1. **KETTLEBELL KG**: Variable

2. **TOTAL SETS**: 3

3. **REST BETWEEN SETS**: 2 Minutes

4. **TOTAL SET LENGTH**: 4 Minutes, 6 Minutes, and 4 Minutes

5. **HAND SWITCHES IN MPH:** 1 to 2 mph

6. **PACE /RPM GOALS**: See RPM Chart / work at fast, slow, and fast pace

7. **EXERCISE SEQUENCE**: Select from any of the 8 core exercises. Stick with the same exercise through the entire sequence. The first set is done at 4 minutes / 2 mph./ LIGHT but working at a fast pace. The second set is done at 6 minutes / 1 hand, working at a slower pace but HEAVY. The last set is done at 4 minutes / 1 to 2 minutes per hand, working at a moderate pace with a moderate weight. Rest 2 minutes between all sets.

HOW THIS WORKOUT DEVELOPED

In the never ending effort to push the envelope, we've found that by using the pyramid principle of light, heavy, moderate, we were able to enhance performance (in your lift of choice) rapidly.

**CLEAN, CLN / PRESS, PR / PUSH PRESS, PP /JERK, JK / LONGCYCLE, L/C / HALF SNATCH, HS / SNATCH, SN / SWING, SW**

ALL PROTOCOLS COPYRIGHTED BY MICHAEL STEFANO 2012

## HIKF CROSS-PERFORMANCE ROUTINE: EXAMPLES

When it comes to combining kettlebells and other fitness modalities, the combinations are endless, and the subject of another book. Below are just a few suggestions on integration that will get you thinking.

### EXAMPLE ONE*

1. JERK  at 6 minutes / 1 mph
2. SQUAT  10 -20
3. SNATCH  at 6 minutes / 1 mph
4. PULL UP  5-10
5. LONGCYCLE  at 6 minutes / 1 mph
6. SIT UP  10-30

*Work within your own range on all exercises

### EXAMPLE TWO*

1. JERK at 4 minutes / 1 mph
2. STEPMILL CLIMBING  30 Floors
3. SNATCH  at 4 minutes / 1 mph
4. TABATA ROWING (interval)  6 minutes
5. LONGCYCLE  at 4 minutes / 1 mph
6. UPHILL TREADMILL WALKING  10 minutes

*Work within your own range on all exercises

### EXAMPLE THREE *

1. LONGCYCLE  at 6 minutes / 1 mph
2. PUSH UP  10-20
3. LONGCYCLE  at 4 minutes / 2 mph
4. SQUAT  10-20
5. LONGCYCLE  at 6 minutes / 1 mph
6. PULLUPS  5-10

*Work within your own range on all exercises*

When developing HIKF Cross Performance routines (integrating traditional exercise with kettlebell fitness movements), the options are almost endless, but certain principles work best.

1. Typically, but not always, kettlebell sets should performed before Cross Performance (CP) work
2. If a recovery period is taken, it is normally before each kettlebell set
3. Kettlebell sets can be seamlessly integrated with resistance or cardiorespiratory exercise
4. CP routines can have a specific focus on a major muscle group (IE: legs, upper body, core)
5. CP routines can have a specific focus on a particular goal (IE: task specific, weight loss, strength)
6. CP routines can be rep-based, or timed, allowing the lifter to work again the clock

# ROUTINE PROGRESSION

New kettlebell lifters should follow the initial 12-Step Progression as a common sense way to get started. Once technique proficiency and general strength conditioning reach a certain level, the lifter should be able to complete all the sets listed above, with the help of the Seven Variables on Intensity. Lifters can progress with one (specific method) or multiple (general method) routines simultaneously. Weight loss is addressed separately.

## GENERAL FITNESS & CONDITIONING

For example, Joe works out five days every week. He performs StrongMan on day one, 20-Minute LongCycle on day two, Crazy 8's on day three, 16-LongCycle Sandwich on day four, and a 10-Minute Mini Q on day five. Each routine is adjusted to the Joe's current level, making sure to provide appropriate intensity, resulting in a challenging workout. The initial routine selection is *adjusted* using the Seven Variables to meet general user goals, while addressing their strengths, as well as limitations. Use this method if your primary goal is health, fitness, or weight loss.

## SPORT OR TASK SPECIFIC

The lifter can take a very different approach from the general fitness progression method, while working on a specific goal, such as improving Snatch technique, or building greater endurance. In the case of working on Snatch technique, the lifter would repeat various Snatch sets from three to five days per week, still adjusting every set using the seven variables, pushing the envelope wherever possible. For the lifter whose main goal is to build a high level of endurance, a logical choice would be to repeat multiple 16 to 20 *Zero Rest Routines*, while moving at a rapid pace (measured in reps per minute [RPM]), each week. Try to match your set sequence to the task at hand. For example, a wrestler who was training for three, six minute rounds, with one minute rest, could do three, six minute sets, with one minute rest, as a way to mimic the actual demand of the match itself.

## WEIGHT LOSS

Weight loss is all about volume, which may, of necessity, limit intensity. Focus mainly on the longer sets, and don't worry too much about how much weight you use. You'll need to keep frequency (how often your train) high as well. Serious weight loss ideally calls for five or six workouts weekly.

# ADDENDUM 1: SAFETY STANDARDS

Kettlebell lifting is serious business. It can be safe, effective, while delivering tremendous results in strength and endurance in a minimalistic, practical setting, but you should always see your health care professional and get medical clearance before starting intense exercise such as High Intensity Kettlebell Fitness.

## SUPERVISION LEVEL

In a professional environment, no lifting of kettlebells should be allowed to go on unsupervised. This is especially true when working with new lifters. An acceptable practice, according to the *World Kettlebell Club,* is to provide one qualified trainer or coach for a maximum of 20 lifters. As a Master Kettlebell Coach for over five years, and owner of a full time kettlebell gym, my personal safety policy doubles this level of supervision to one coach or trainer for every ten lifters when working with *inexperienced* lifters.

Kettlebell trainers must maintain *continuous* supervision over all lifting. Trainers shall be sure to position themselves so as to maintain a clear view of the entire facility and all lifters. The trainer must constantly monitor and enforce rules, ensure proper technique is being adhered to, while being ever vigilant for unsafe conditions that may arise. During any type of break, when there are no kettlebell trainers maintaining vigilant supervision over all lifters, no movement of the kettlebell should occur.

## DESIGNATED LIFTING AREA

In addition, kettlebell lifters should work in *designated lifting areas* only. An area of at least 5 feet (side to side) by 7 feet (front to back) should be maintained around an active lifter. Ideally this designated area should be marked by use of a *raised platform* or *lifting mat*.

TRAFFIC FLOW

For safe entrance and exit, there should be a walkway of 36 inches maintained through the lifting area that doesn't encumber the lifter, which also provides a clear path to the exit. No lifting should occur in this area, especially when students / lifters are moving in and out of the facility.

Below is a summary of the 4 most important safety points.

1.  Maintain an adequate level of supervision, minimally 1 coach or trainer for every 20 lifters

2.  Maintain a safe distance around each lifter, minimally 5 ft (side to side) by 7 ft (front to back)

3.  Maintain a designated lifting area for all lifters, clearly marked, or use a raised mat or platform

4.  Provide a clear path of at least 36 inches to all entrance and exits from the lifting area

## DISCLAIMER

This is the PERSONAL / HOME version of the High Intensity Kettlebell Fitness (HIKF) Book by Michael Stefano, intended for nonprofessional use only. To purchase the professional version of this course, go to: kbgym.com . This book is part of the American Council on Exercise *approved* KBNY High Intensity Kettlebell Fitness Trainer Course.

See your doctor, and get clearance before performing any of the exercises contained in this book.

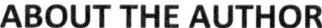

# ABOUT THE AUTHOR

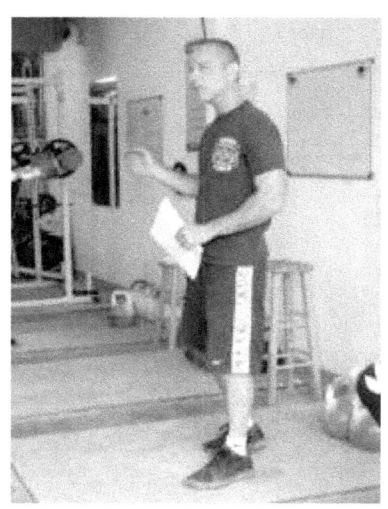

Mike Stefano is a retired NYC Fire Captain and author of The Firefighter's Workout Book, published by HarperCollins in October 2000. The Firefighter's Workout has sold over 60,000 copies world-wide. In 2007, Mr. Stefano was appointed the Fire Rescue Advisor for the American Kettlebell Club, and studied closely with Russian world champion, Valery Fedorenko - working side by side with Coach Fedorenko. Coach Stefano was instrumental in the initial development of the American Kettlebell Club. Today, Mike owns and operates KBNY, using his High Intensity Kettlebell Fitness and Cross-Performance Training to develop android levels of strength and endurance, while literally transforming you into a fat burning machine. He works with people from all walks of life from accountants to firefighter candidates, and everything in between. Coach Stefano offers a Kettlebell Trainer Course that is American Council on Exercise (ACE) approved, as well as a brand new High Intensity Kettlebell Fitness eBook. You can find out more about Coach Stefano on Facebook, Twitter, YouTube or his website, www.**kbgym.com.**